Healthy Living
When You're Over 50

(50 is the new 20)

David Boothway

DEDICATION

To my wonderful wife, Jeanette, and lovely daughters, Kerry and Kirsten, who taught me what real health is.

CONTENTS

ACKNOWLEDGMENTS

Inspiration for writing this book came from my family. They are great at encouraging me to live my dream. Thanks to family, friends and my grammar guru who gave me honest comments and feedback on the drafts. You all made the journey fun and enjoyable.

1 THE START OF MY JOURNEY

This book is written to inspire you to live a healthy life. To be energised and full of life. To be your own health hero. It is tailored for all ages but leans towards those who are about midway through their life and are wondering how to live the next 50 years feeling better than the previous 50 years. None of us wants a body that is riddled with sickness, as we can't then enjoy life. No one wants to live in pain, full of misery, kept alive with heart bypass surgery, stents and medication that punishes our internal organs. I am sure you are like me, wanting quality of life as well as length of days, so we can enjoy life with our grandchildren and fill life with beauty, joy and happiness.

This book is based on my own personal journey to a healthier me after I became 50. In my younger days, I believed that my body was highly resilient to whatever I ate. I believed I could eat anything, and my body would select what it wanted and discharge the rest. When I ate a burger, I believed my body would digest it, pick out what nutrients it needed and get rid of the toxins and bad stuff. Little did I know I was poisoning my body.

The same went for my external body. If I got a cut, I figured my body would repair it properly. If it was sunburnt after a day in the surf, I would be sore for a day or two, but I believed my body fully healed itself. Little did I know I was so wrong.

The same principle applied mentally as well. I would pride myself in studying all night with no sleep.

I was active – I loved the outdoors. Hiking, running, canoeing, tennis, surfing—I loved it all. My body seemed to be inherently capable of sustained physical activity, with almost no training.

But turning 50 has given me a different perspective and a wiser outlook.

I have friends, who were like me, but now have cancer. My dad died too early. My mom has diabetes. Heart attacks, strokes and Alzheimer's is ravaging our family's friendship circle. Something is seriously wrong.

Three years ago, my daughter became a vegan. It triggered me to find out more about health. It taught me to look at all aspects of my life through a better lens.

At 50+, I am now healthier than ever. But I am not perfect, and I am always learning.

Hopefully, these insights will help you.

This book covers the four health pillars of food, exercise, wisdom, and stress management.

This is a short compact book full of insights, podcasts and website links, videos, book recommendations and a free health chart.

I like to remind my daughters that for us older healthy folk, 50 is the new 20.

Yours in 50+ health,

David Boothway

2 BE YOUR OWN HERO

"If you look inside yourself, and you believe, you can be your own hero." **Mariah Carey**

Be your own health hero. Feel empowered by taking control of your own health. Find new likeminded people who are also health-conscious. Some of your old friends may think you are weird, but remember that good health is not weird. It is great. Not everyone sees the light at the same time.

As you work your way through your health journey, find solutions that work for you and share your story with others.

Being healthy is 90% mind muscle and 10% physical muscle. When you know you should not order French fries, it is not your body that physically wants them; it's your mind. Become your own hero and learn to master your mind. Heroes make a difference. Neil Armstrong become a hero when he took one small step on the moon. Be your own hero when you take one small step towards your own better health. Be a hero each week as you move forward.

This mindset creates great forward momentum. Entertain yourself with laughter to keep your journey light and enjoyable. Surprise yourself. Be your own health hero so you can enjoy the riches of life; happiness, joy and love. Play it forward. Allow it to inspire someone else.

Share your health hero journey.

3 FOOD: YOUR BEST FRIEND OR WORST FOE

**"Let food be thy medicine and medicine be thy food."
Hippocrates**

Love your food. It is what keeps you alive. What is the point of eating what you do not like or starving yourself? That is just plain stupid.

Having said that, we need to understand that our culture, and what we have trained our taste buds to like, determines what we eat. I remember I used to hate the taste of mushrooms. Now I love them.

So here is the secret: Retrain your taste buds to crave what is good for you. It is transformational and easier than you think.

In simple terms, you need to train your tongue to love plant-based food. Medical and health sciences now show, beyond any shadow of doubt, that a plant-based diet is the healthiest by far.

Weird is no doubt your first response. It was mine too. Emotionally, my brain was telling me, "Hell no. Meat is king."

It took a lot to convince me. I resisted for many months. In fact, I insisted that my vegan daughter eat meat for protein. Margret Mead said it so well: "It is easier to change a man's religion than change his diet."

So here is the answer: You need to put emotion aside. Put

culture aside. Put slick corporate marketing aside. Put aside lobby groups that are funded millions by multinational corporates to create laws and guidelines that reinforce poor health. Put confusing media mixed messages aside. Remember, even doctors smoked at one stage and advertised cigarettes. The same happens now. Most doctors and nutritionists love meat, eggs and dairy and therefore promote it.

The truth is, we need to get down to facts. Be objective and not emotional about the truth. Seek the whole truth about nutrition and health, not half-truths. The facts tell us we don't need meat in our diet. In fact, eating meat will degrade our health. Processed meat, like bacon, is as bad for you as smoking. The UN classifies processed meat as a class-one carcinogen; it is in the same class as asbestos. Animal foods, such as meat, dairy and eggs, are the major causes of sicknesses, such as heart disease, strokes, and cancers.

So, where do we get our protein, nutrients and vitamins? The answer is through plants, which is the same place cattle get it from. Cattle are simply an inefficient middleman. Plus, the meat carries a whole lot of hidden nasties, like antibiotics, growth hormones and many dangerous diseases.

At this point, it is worth your time to watch two health documentaries:

1. Dr McGregor's 2016 YouTube video *'How Not to Die'*
2. *'What the health'* released in 2017

So, how can you create a plant-based diet that is healthy, price competitive, convenient and appealing to your taste buds? This is a good question. I found the easiest way is to do the following:

1. Try a plant-based lifestyle for 21 days. If you like it, then continue; if not, go back to your old ways. I found the 21-day Kick Starter by PCRM to be the best. It is easy and has great recipes and lots of nutritional information. Go to www.pcrm.org and search for 21-day kickstart.

2. Remove all meat, dairy and egg foods out of your fridge and pantry, and dump them in the bin. (Obviously, you can't do this if not everyone in your household is migrating towards better health. If you can, treat meat, dairy and egg addiction like alcohol addiction—don't have easy access to it.)

3. Replace all these products with plant-based equivalents, such as almond or rice milk instead of dairy milk. Stock up with dairy-free yoghurt, dairy-free ice cream, plant-based "meat" burgers, plant-based "chicken" strips, and plant-based "meat" pies. Use a plant-based recipe book or the internet if you are unsure what to use. My wife makes the most delicious meringues from chickpeas. They taste and look the same. You would never guess they were not made from egg whites.

4. Dump all junk food in the bin. Fill your kitchen with fresh vegetables and fruit. The golden rule is the less processed the food, the better for your health.

5. Get yourself a plant-based recipe book or google the millions of plant-based recipes online. I love the Revive cookbooks by Jeremy Dixon. For great free online recipes, go to the website *Forks over Knives*.

6. Get yourself a set of go-to plant-based recipes of your favourite meals. If you like lasagne, try lots of plant-based lasagne recipes until you find one you like. Sometimes it is as easy as replacing an animal product with a plant product. For instance, try replacing dairy milk with rice milk in a pancake mixture.

7. Stock up with go-to healthy snacks. If you are like me, you love nibbling between meals. I love snacks. If you don't have good snacks, the temptation to binge on junk snacks is high.

8. When eating out at a café or restaurant, you will find you need to be creative to modify an existing meal (such as request they leave off the dairy cheese). Often, the chef will love to create a great plant-based dish that looks and tastes amazing—all you have to do is ask. A lot of Eastern cuisine has plant-based dishes. Ask for your coffee with almond milk, or better still, select an herbal tea without milk.

9. Keep hydrated. You need about 8 glasses of water a day. Coffee and tea counts, but always remember water is best. Remember, all your plant-based food has high water content, so include this in your water count.

10. Eat fibre; it promotes a healthy gut, keeps you regular, mitigates diseases like colon cancer, and helps remove toxins out of your body. Fibre is in all plant-based foods but it is not in meat.

Be your hero on this journey. Is this an easy journey? For some, it is. It all depends how convinced you are deep down. Some transition over 6 months. Some start with meatless Mondays. Some switch in a day. There is no fixed rule. It all depends how much you really want good health. It is your choice, your journey. Also remember not to ridicule others who don't change as fast as you. We each need to embrace the path we have chosen.

Will you stumble sometimes? For sure. All heroes stumble. Don't worry. Like learning to ride a bike, dust yourself off, get back on and enjoy the journey. You have years of cultural food baggage that you are dealing with. Plus, the media creates confusing messages (on purpose to sell more bad food, papers and magazines), so you are bombarded every day with seemingly conflicting messages. This tends to result in a confused social norm for society. And a confused society keeps doing the same thing it always does, which is exactly what the big corporations want so they can keep you hooked on their bad products. More sales equals more profits. This in turn keeps the shareholders happy. Is it not ironic that our pension funds probably have shares in companies that make bad food that makes us sick, and shares in hospitals and pharmaceutical companies that we go to help make us better. Surely, it is better for society to eat better and not get sick in the first place.

The Blue Zone study, supported by National Geographic, investigate people who live longer and better. Have a look at their website or look at Dan Beuttner's TED Talk "How to live to be a 100+".

You may ask, are there any foods that we should eat daily that are the best to eat? The best list I have found is one by Dr. McGreger. He lists the following superfoods: beans (3 servings a day), berries (1 serving a day), other fruit (servings a day) , cruciferous vegetables (1 serving a day), greens (2 servings a day), other vegetables (2 servings a day), flaxseeds (1 serving a day), nuts (1 serving a day), spices , whole grains (3 servings a day). He has the list on a smart phone App called Daily Dozen.

Love being your own food hero.

4 EXERCISE

"To walk in nature is to witness a thousand miracles."
Mary Davis

We are born to move, yet modern day technology has made us slothful. We sit in a car, sit in the office, sit at home in front of the TV and then lie down to sleep. Our body craves mobility and physical work but our daily routine is giving it the opposite, and it is killing us. Research shows that we need at least 90 minutes of moderate activity a day to be healthy. Wow, I hear you say, that is a lot. Yes, it seems like a lot to our sedate lifestyles.

The trick is to look for activity in your normal day.

Your daily exercise needs to be made up of formal and informal activities. Formal is where you have your daily exercise routine, such as a walk in the morning. Informal is where you use the stairs instead of the lift at work.

Here are a few tips I have found useful:
1. Start small. If you are overweight and have never jogged before then start out with a walk to the end of your block and back. Do that for five days.
2. Steadily increase. Start small but steadily increase your exercise to a good level. Increase the distance to include a few

more street blocks the next week. Soon, your body will crave the outdoor walk. That's good. In the end, you want to get to the stage where you are having at least 30 minutes of aerobic activity.

3. <u>Choose an activity you enjoy.</u> If it is tennis, then play good strong tennis for at least 30 minutes.

4. <u>Walk or jog with a friend,</u> if possible. This creates a mutual obligation to not fail each other; therefore, the routine is more likely to be upheld. Plus, it is great to catch up and have a chat while walking/jogging/working out at the gym.

5. <u>Do 30 minutes aerobic activity.</u> Slowly build up week on week to a 30-minute activity. After six months of steadily increasing your workout, you want to be at 30 minutes of aerobic activity per day, 5 days a week. Your total daily activity (formal and informal) should lean towards 90 minutes a day.

6. <u>If you miss a day, don't torture yourself,</u> and don't try to catch up. Don't do double the next day. Simply pick up where you left off. We all miss days due to sickness or a busy work day. That is part of normal life.

You may wish to know what my daily routine is. I am a morning person, so I love to get up early at sunrise. For me, it is the best time of the day. It is crisp and I can listen to the birds calling; it is an opportunity for me to be at one with myself and my God while out on my run. In summer, I go for a morning jog, about 3 km, during which I do a few exercises at a local park playground. Then I cycle to work (about 18 km round trip). At work, I walk the stairs (I work on the 4th floor) and I love to walk around the city block at lunch to clear my head. After getting home after work, my wife and I walk the dogs for about half an hour, which is also a good time to catch up on the day's happenings.

Each of us have different circumstances, so through trial and error, you will find a daily routine that works for you. Don't feel obligated to copy mine.

Keep exercise simple and fun. My routine works for me. I enjoy it. You may find it easier to jog at your lunch break, or you may be a gym person and fit that in after work. I do not belong to a gym, fitness club, or sports club, but making the gym a regular part of your routine would be beneficial for those who do belong, as this creates a great exercise discipline. Team sports lift the soul as well.

One of the key things to remember is that you do not need the latest gizmos, smartest shoes, or best fashion fitness clothes to get fit. Often, we use the excuse that we don't have the latest mod cons, so we don't exercise. The beauty about exercise is that it does not have to be expensive. You can jog along a beach barefoot, swim in a 20-year-old swimsuit, or exercise at a public playground. You don't need a $1000 watch that counts steps, or a $5000 bike, or belong to an expensive gym. My running shoes and bike are both bottom of the range and now 10 years old. I love looking at my running shoes in the morning as I put them on. They are a bit tattered and torn with a hole near the big toe. They remind me of the wonderful journey we have been on together, beautiful places we have seen, and lovely people we have met. My advice is to spend less time worrying about what you wear and more time being active.

The beauty about exercise is that it is portable. I love that I can go away on business and go for morning jogs in a new city because all I need to do is pack my jogging shoes and some light jogging clothes.

Be strict with yourself and keep exercise regular, but also be flexible and adapt as the seasons change. Recently, I moved to a city located in a colder climate, and I found this made it harder for morning exercise. We all look for excuses, don't we? It is important we do our best to overcome these minor human frailties. I need to learn to be flexible and do my summer morning routine in the afternoon in winter when it is warmer. Our goal is health, not excuses.

As I have gotten older, I have found I need more discipline to do exercise. If it rains, I don't exercise. Maybe I am getting soft as I get older. If it rains, I sometimes do an inside routine, but I would be lying if I said this was regular.

It is important to be active whenever you can; mow the lawn

(don't get someone else to do it), paint the walls yourself, wash the dishes (don't load the dishwasher), wash your car (don't take it to a drive-thru washer), clean your own house (don't hire a cleaner), make yourself a veggie garden (good exercise and good food without pesticides), and walk your neighbour's dog.

The point is to enjoy putting one step in front of the other.

Enjoy being your own exercise hero.

5 SEEK WISDOM

"Blessed is the man who finds wisdom." Proverbs 3:13

Wisdom is a like a golden sunset: it enriches your soul. Wisdom is not head knowledge. Wisdom is about cultivating a hunger to learn more about what is good and implementing the best.

Be your own wisdom hero.

Sometimes, we feel overloaded with all the knowledge being pushed on us each day. Last week, I counted over 120 magazines at our local food supermarket. The amount is crazy, isn't it? Add on the daily papers, TV news and social media and it is no wonder we feel confused. We are being bombarded with information that has no lasting value.

To keep sane, we need to develop filters to keep the noise out.

Here are some tips I currently use:

1. Be the captain of what comes into your body. Choose what media you want to look at regularly each day. At present, my daily wisdom routine includes the following:
    1.1. Listening to two chapters of the Bible while I eat breakfast. I love listening to the Message Bible through the YouVersion free Bible app.

1.2. Listening to a wisdom podcast while I cycle to and back from work. My favourites at the moment are the podcasts of Rob Bell and Rich Roll.

1.3. Reading the daily paper for 10 minutes while having my morning tea at work.

1.4. Reading a non-fiction book for 20 minutes at lunch.

1.5. Glancing at my home emails for 10 minutes when I get home.

1.6. Limiting my TV news intake to no more than 20 minutes each night (even though I love watching it). If I am really disciplined, I don't watch TV.

1.7. Reading from a book before I sleep.

1.8. Currently, I am trying a social media cleanse. I try not to look at Facebook or Instagram. I do not have Twitter or Snapchat accounts, and I visit LinkedIn about once every 6 months. My time on social media probably adds up to about half an hour over a month.

2. Cultivate a desire to learn good stuff. Hold the world media at arm's length because if you are not careful, it will saturate you with nothing but gossip and ill information. I like to actively learn each day; it keeps me sharp and my cognitive brain active.

3. Be flexible enough to lean into a better way but strong enough not to be fickle and be swayed by each new wind. I have found that truths have a good base note. They are foundation material that is stable. It does not need corporate hype to keep it standing.

4. Try practicing the art of long, deep conversations. I have found this profoundly inspirational in our "once over lightly" world of quick-fix addictions. Practice this at the dinner table or have a hearty conversation with an elderly person at church or at a social gathering; their wisdom is infectious, and their mistakes and things that went well will have you rolling with laughter. You will have a new wise best friend and new-found wisdom.

5. Try making friends with your library again. Read a book (not an electronic one) for an hour before sleeping. This is a habit you will never regret.

Be your own wisdom hero.

6 STRESS MANAGEMENT

"Never underestimate the importance of removing stuff you don't need." Joshua Becker

Stress management is important for good health. It reduces blood pressure, thus lowering the risk of heart attack or stroke. It reduces the release of cortisone, which is the hormone that increases the hardening of the arteries, and amongst other things, it reduces the possibility of getting stomach ulcers. With good stress management, you will sleep better and have a better quality and length of life.

I personally have found stress management the hardest health attribute to master. Maybe that is because stress management is best achieved through a collective of actions, not just one. Also, I find that stress comes from different directions (such as work, family, natural disasters, finance, death of someone close), and it feels like it comes in batches. I find I am stressed the most when events outside my control affect my family, friends and staff. For instance, I dislike the bad things that happen, beyond my control to loyal staff who are bullied or treated in a dehumanising manner due to corporate powerplays.

Stressful events have also taught me a lot. For instance, the extreme inner pain I felt during the death of my father has given me the ability to be alongside others who experience similar pain. I can now empathise with others in an area where previously I only had intellectual knowledge. I have grown to appreciate that you can only truly "love your neighbour" when you can empathise alongside them.

Stress comes in all shapes and sizes. Here are some of the best ways I have found to destress:

1. Cherish your family. They are a gift from God. Serve them more, love them more, tell them you love them, and spend more time with them. Put your love words into action. Doing family stuff is a great de-stressor. I love going for an easy cruiser bicycle ride with my daughter around our neighbourhood.

2. Exercise. Working out regularly is one of the best ways to relax your body and mind.

3. Deep breathing. This cleans out your lungs and fills you with fresh air. Breathe in deeply for a count of 5. Hold your breath for a count of 3. Let your breath out for a count of 10. Repeat three times. I find it good practice to do this first thing in morning, at lunch and in the evening.

4. Eat well. Seek out a plant-based diet. Avoid smoking, coffee, drugs and other addictive or stress-enhancing substances.

5. Slow down and don't fill your day with too many things. We live in a fast-paced world, and I used to think that a full fast-paced day was good. It gave me a sense of accomplishment. But I have realised that it is more meaningful and less stressful to take the slow and steady route. This may sound patronising, but learn to say no in a nice way, both to others and to yourself.

6. Take a break. The natural cycles of nature teach us to take breaks. Night and day, high and low tide, the four seasons, the principle of the Sabbath (a time for reflection)—use these

principles during the day as well. Create breaks, seasons and times of reflection. Take time to recharge your batteries. Taking time to "sharpen the saw" is a principle that Stephen Covey teaches. We can hack all day with a blunt saw and get little done, even though we have expended much energy. Take a break to sharpen the saw; fill your mind with a better way to enable you to achieve twice as much after the break.

7. Talk about your problems. We all have problems, often in the categories of relationships, work, family, friends, finance and health. Each week, a different problem may surface. If we bottle up the problems in our mind, they can become all-consuming. We toss and turn at night, sleep less, and wake up grumpy and more stressed. Find a trustworthy person you can speak to, or chat to a counsellor. Talking does not necessarily take the problem away, but it helps reduce the stress.

8. Help others. Often, when we feel stressed and down in the dumps, a good remedy is to help the less fortunate. Mow the lawn for a neighbour who is sick, help out at a charity shop, visit a sick friend in the hospital. Give others your empathy. When I lost my father, I was very stressed as I had changed between jobs two weeks earlier and was still in the process of changing cities. I am now able to draw on that experience, remember the depth of my pain and be alongside others when they are in a similar need and time of stress.

9. Make time for hobbies. This is "me" time. Find out what you really enjoy, such as fishing, sewing, tennis, rock climbing, and cooking. Now, cut yourself time to do it regularly. Your absorption into your hobby will help destress your mind.

10. Practice yoga and meditation. Join a class or undertake the free online 30 Days of Yoga course with Adriene. For those who are stiff and inflexible like me, try doing these classes with your daughters. The lounge will be filled with laughter.

11. Spend time with your god. Pray. Read. Meditate. Contribute. Share. Give. Love. Practice grace. Forgive often. These are all easier said than done, but such is our walk to a higher spiritual life. It is good to remember that, like Jacob, often when we have been with God, we walk with a limp. It

reminds us to cherish humility and to remember we have weaknesses and so do others. Don't expect perfection for yourself or others. Genuine quiet time with God will generate your deepest tranquility. Psalm 23 reads, "Even though I walk through the valley of the shadow of death, I will fear no evil, for thou art with me."

12. Align with your purpose. Each morning, ask yourself two questions: Who am I? What am I doing here? Connect with your god to help you with direction and meaning. This will give you significant inner peace. This feels easy when life is good but hard when you are in the middle of trauma, your walls are falling down and your inner peace is knocked off the perch. That's a signal to look deep inside again to reaffirm and realign your purpose. My daughter has this good phase: "You have to work for your own dream; otherwise, you work for someone else's dream."

13. Touch nature. Reconnect with the natural circadian rhythm of the earth. Lie outside on the lawn flat on your back. Look at the blue sky or stars. Close your eyes and reconnect. Our cities have pushed nature far away. They are filled with litter, concrete, tar roads and noise. They have piped rivers underground to build shopping malls on top. Our bodies crave to be reconnected to nature. So, try something like walking barefoot on the beach. Wade barefoot through a stream. Touch and smell a wildflower while on your walk. Feel the soil in your hands as you work in your veggie patch.

14. Learn to live with less. We have been trained to consume and want more—another shirt, the latest mobile phone, a new car. We feel stressed when we see others possessing the things we want. In essence, we are coveting. The old wisdom teachings, like the Bible, say that happiness is not found in owning more stuff. Learning to live with less is hard in a world that pushes you to want more. Debt reduction is a great stress reliever. Read some books or watch a documentary on living with less. A good place to start is to visit Joshua Becker's website *Becoming Minimalist*. Also google "minimalism," "waste is for tossers," or "tiny house" or search for these phrases on YouTube. Living with less means you stress less about paying the next bill, about tidying your

room, and about keeping stuff clean and serviced. It frees up time, money, and brain space. It allows you the freedom to do the things you really enjoy, such as spending time with those you love.

15. Keep a stress journal. Sometimes, when our minds are so full, we don't know where to start to destress. Try this simple technique. Each day, try writing down what you feel stressed about in your journal. (My daughter introduced me to keeping a journal of thoughts, notes and ideas, and now I love it.) After a few days, you should see a pattern or a few common themes. Now, try to address one or two. Use the principles listed above to help. Over time, as each stress point is reduced or eliminated, you will move towards a more harmonic you.

Enjoy the journey to a better mental wellbeing and a better you.

Love yourself and be your own harmonic hero.

7 REBORN

Be reborn to newness of life

The best times in life come after you experience an epiphany and are reborn. Burying your old unhealthy habits is a rebirth to a new you. A healthier you.

Being reborn is all around us. Nature is full of examples. Each dawn is the birth of a new day. A caterpillar rebirths into a butterfly. Rebirths create the beauty that is around us. Your health rebirth will create a beautiful you.

"How do I become reborn?" you may ask. Start with a commitment to yourself. Try saying these words: "From today, I will put aside all prejudices and seek to experience the joy of new health." Ask for spiritual support from your god.

Tell others of your joy. Tell them that you are seeking out a new healthier you. Ask them for encouragement and support and to hold you accountable.

Photostat the Health Reminder sheet and score yourself each day. It gives you your benchmark and a line in the sand from which you move forward.

For inspiration, watch the short documentary on YouTube *November Project: Showing Up*.

The wise saying holds true: "A journey of a 1000 miles starts with one step." That first step is your rebirth. Now comes the continuous learning, the doing and the enjoyment of knowing you have started something good.

Ignite the health hero in you.

Be your own reborn health hero.

8 HEALTHY LIVING CHART

A free Healthy Living wall chart located on the next page is included as a useful tool. Print it out and stick it up on your bathroom mirror, fridge door, notice board or in your journal. I put mine on my study notice board and in the front cover of my journal. It is a checklist and a simple reminder of the important things to do each day to be healthy.

It keeps things simple and easy.

Make a promise to yourself today that each new day, you will live healthier than the last.

See it as a journey and enjoy the ride. Health is not a destination. Health is a living, doing thing.

In the process, become your own health hero. The outcomes of joy, happiness and loving yourself are yours for the taking.

Healthy Living: Daily Reminder

Health Hero	Today I felt like a health hero	
	I am enjoying my health journey	
Food	I enjoy what I eat	
	I eat plant-based food	
	My snacks and treats are wholesome	
	I drink water (4 to 8 glasses/day)	
Exercise	I make my everyday life active	
	I take active breaks every 30 min	
	I do at least 30 min of aerobic activity each day	
	My activities are fun	
	I do yoga/stretch	
Seek wisdom	I listen actively	
	I read wise words (15min per day)	
	I actively help others	
	Social media is used rarely	
	I nurture my spiritual life (read, pray, meditate)	
	I actively learn each day (15 min per day)	
Reduce Stress	I breathe deeply (3 x a day)	
	I talk to trustworthy people about my stress issues	
	I actively nurture and love my family	
	I take micro breaks and walk	
	I slow down and respectfully say no	
	I actively make my life simpler and less cluttered	
Reborn	Each day, I am reborn into living healthier	

Healthy Living (50 is the new 20) © David Boothway

David Boothway

9 USEFUL RESOURCES

These are a few great resources based on the Less is More principle.

May I suggest you start with watching the "Forks Over Knives" documentary, then look at the "How Not To Die" 2016 video by Dr. McGregor. Both are on YouTube. After that watch the "What Makes a Good Life? Lessons From The Longest Study on Happiness." Ted talk by Robert Waldinger.

Websites
- www.nutritionfacts.org Best website for factual nutritional information plus good advice on exercise
- www.forksoverknives.com Great health and great recipes
- www.becomingminimalist.com Stress free living
- www.yogawithadriene.com/30days/   Easy and fun yoga
- www.ediblebackyard.co.nz Growing great food in small spaces.

Food recipes
www.forksoverknives.com
www.pcrm.org/health   Great 21 day kickstarter programme for better eating

Podcasts
Rich Roll (Great interviews with experts in health and wellbeing)
Rob Bell (Spiritual interviews and wisdom thinking like that found in the Bible.)

Apps
YouVersion – Bible (Many versions of Bible plus great audio bible)
Daily Dozen – top superfoods – daily check
21 Day Veg Kickstart (plant based recipes for 21 days)

YouTube clips
- Best beginner body weight workouts. Exercise at park or at home. https://www.youtube.com/watch?v=uPFgNEKxMds
- How to start Calisthenics – Complete Guide (Beginners). The video clip gives good beginner tips and also links to more advanced exercises in the notes below the video clip. https://www.youtube.com/watch?v=uJ9rAUQhM2g
- 'November Project : Showing Up' an inspirational video on keeping healthy and helping others.

Documentaries (Look on YouTube or Netflix)
- Dr. McGregor's 2016 YouTube video "How Not To Die"
- Forks over Knives   (Reversing heart attacks with diet)
- Whatthehealth (Better health though diet, not popping pills.)
- Cowspiracy (Living a diet in harmony with the environment)

Ted Talks
- Why I Lived a Zero Waste Life – Lauren Zinger
- What Makes a Good Life? Lessons from the longest study on happiness – Robert Waldinger.
- How to live to 100+ by Dan Buettner. Lessons from people who have live longer, better.

Books
- The Revive Café Cookbook by Jeremy Dixon – Delicious, healthy & easy recipes.
- Enjoying the Bible by H A Whittaker – great simple reading that makes wisdom teaching come alive.

ABOUT THE AUTHOR

David Boothway is a professional engineer with a master's degree. He calls himself a reborn engineer, one that uses engineering to restore cities to living places and restore the earth's ecosystems. Why? Because he loves uplifting the wellbeing of society and establishing true multigenerational prosperity. In essence, to use our collective talents to be good stewards of our precious earth and families. He loves the beauty of the Christian faith and freely admits he falls short of its high calling. His wife, Jeanette, inspires him and keeps him grounded. They have been blessed with two lovely daughters. Born in the United Kingdom, he has lived in Kenya, South Africa, and now in New Zealand. He loves the outdoors and tries to surf and play tennis. After reaching 50, his daughters taught him how to eat and live better. He recently gave a Ted Talk entitled "Finding our Stolen Rivers."

www.ingramcontent.com/pod-product-compliance
Lightning Source LLC
Chambersburg PA
CBHW061935280526
45787CB00004B/1610